Mediterranean Meal recipes for a fit lifestyle

*Fuel your day
with balanced Mediterranean
flavors and savors*

Lana Green

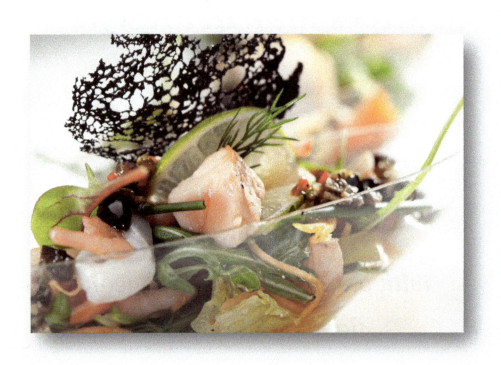

Table of Contents

Mushroom & Cardamom, Squash Soup

Prep Time: 8 min

Cook Time: 30 min

Serve: 3

Ingredients:

- 1 tsp ginger

- One leek

- 1 tsp Celtic sea salt

- 125 ml of coconut cream

- 200 g mushrooms

- 250 ml passata

- 300 ml of water

- 350g of peeled squash

- Four cardamom pods

- 1 cup herbs

- Dash of coconut oil

Preparation:

1. In a bowl, sugar, milk, salt, ginger, and past, cardamom into a squash. Cook and for 15 minutes. Blend the mixture.

2. Sauté mushrooms in heated oil for five minutes. Serve in serving dish by making layers and serve.

Pomegranate Avocado Salsa

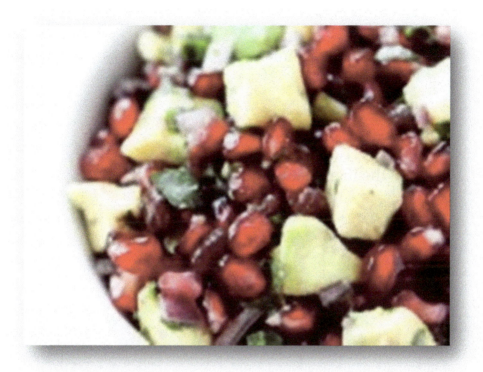

Prep Time: 10 min

Cook Time: 10 min

Serve: 6

Ingredients:

- 1/3 cup red onion diced

- 1/3 cup chopped cilantro

- Two pomegranates sliced

- One jalapeno chopped

- One avocado

- the juice of 1 lime

- 1 tsp sea salt

Preparation:

Mix all the ingredients and serve.

White Bean Bruschetta

Prep Time: 5 min

Cook Time: 10min

Serve: 6

Ingredients:

- 1 -2 clove garlic sliced
- 1 cup cannellini beans, cooked
- ½ tsp red pepper flakes
- 2 tbsp balsamic vinegar
- 2 tbsp olive oil
- 2 tbsp basil leaves
- 6 slices Italian bread
- garlic
- Salt to taste
- Pepper to taste

Preparation:

Mix all the items in a jar except bread. Toast the bread and spread the mixture, and serve.

Baked Fish Fillets

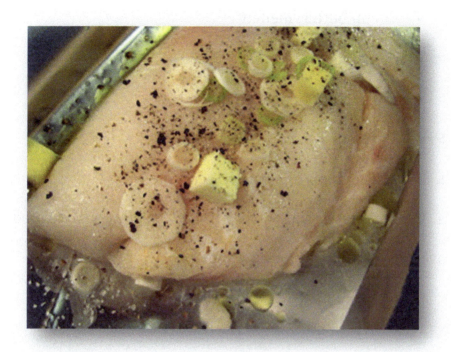

Prep Time: 10 min

Cook Time: 20 min

Serve: 6

Ingredients:

- 2 tbsp lemon juice

- 2 lb mackerel fillets

- 1 tsp salt

- 1 tbsp vegetable oil

- ¼ cup butter, melted

- ⅛ tsp paprika

- ⅛ tsp black pepper

Preparation:

1. Mix all the items in a bowl except fillets.

2. Coat fillets with the mixture and bake in a preheated oven at 350 degrees for 25 minutes.

Black Bean-Salmon Stir-Fry

Prep Time: 5 min

Cook Time: 20 min

Serve: 4

Ingredients:

- 2 tsp cornstarch

- 2 tbsp rice vinegar

- 2 tbsp sauce black bean garlic

- 12 oz mung bean sprouts

- 1 tbsp canola oil

- 1 tbsp rice wine

- 1 lb salmon

- One pinch of red pepper

- 1 cup diced scallions

- ¼ cup of water

Preparation:

1. Mix all the ingredients except salmon and set aside. The sauce is ready. Cook salmon in heated oil for three minutes from each side.

2. Add the sauce to salmon and cook for a minute. Mix in scallions and beans and cook for five minutes.

Michael Symon's Grilled Salmon and Zucchini Salad

Prep Time: 8 min

Cook Time: 8 min

Serves: 4

Ingredients:

- ¼ cup chopped fresh dill

- ¼ cup sliced almonds, toasted

- ½ tsp black pepper, divided

- ¾ tsp kosher salt, divided

- One lemon

- 3 cups sliced zucchini

- 3 tbsp olive oil, divided

- 24 oz salmon fillets

Preparation:

1. Coat fillets with salt, pepper, and oil and grill over a preheated grill for five minutes for each side.

2. Transfer in a plate. Mix all the remaining ingredients and pour over fillets.

Grilled Salmon with Mustard & Herbs

Prep Time: 5 min

Cook Time: 40 min

Serve: 4

Ingredients:

- ¼ tsp salt

- One clove garlic

- 1 lb salmon

- 1 tbsp Dijon mustard

- Two lemons sliced

- 30 sprigs mixed herbs

Preparation:

1. Arrange a layer of lemon followed by herbs on a baking tray. Mix garlic with salt and coat over salmon.

2. Place the salmon on herbs. Place the pan in the grill and cook for 25 minutes.

Herb-Baked Fish Fillets

Prep Time: 15 min

Cook Time: 15 min

Serve: 4

Ingredients:

- Kosher salt to taste

- Black pepper to taste

- 2 tbsp butter

- 1/4 tsp dried thyme

- 1/4 cup corn flakes

- 1/4 cup of Onion

- 1/2 tsp dried tarragon

- 1 tsp chopped parsley

- 1 tbsp melted butter

- 1 lb fish fillets

- One clove garlic (minced)

Preparation:

3.1. Sauté garlic, onions, thyme, and tarragon in heated butter for two minutes. Transfer the mixture over fish fillets.

2. Lightly sauté corn in butter and sprinkle salt and pepper to make cornflake crumbs.

3. Bake the fillets in an oven at 450 degrees for 15 minutes.

Japanese Salmon & Soba Noodle Salad

Prep Time: 10 min

Cook Time: 10 min

Serve: 4

Ingredients:

- 1/2 tbsp rice vinegar

- 1 tsp soy sauce

- 2 tbsp canola oil

- 2 tsp sesame oil

- 200 g snow peas sliced

- 250 g soba noodles

- Three salmon fillets

- Four green onions sliced

- 60 g baby spinach leaves

Preparation:

1. Bake the fillets wrapped in foil in a preheated oven at 180 degrees for five minutes. Cook peas in boiling water for about 2 minutes and drain them.

2. Now cook noodles in the same water for five minutes.

3. Now mix everything in a bowl and serve.

Walnut-rosemary crusted salmon

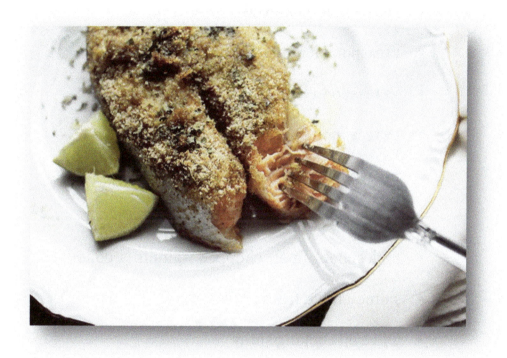

Prep Time: 15 min

Cook Time: 0 min

Serve: 4

Ingredients:

- teaspoons Dijon mustard

- ¼ teaspoon lemon zest

- 1 teaspoon chopped fresh rosemary

- ¼ teaspoon of crushed red pepper

- 1 clove garlic, minced

- 1 teaspoon lemon juice

- ½ teaspoon honey

- ½ teaspoon kosher salt

- 1 teaspoon extra-virgin olive oil

- tablespoons panko breadcrumbs

- tablespoons finely chopped walnuts (1 pound)

- salmon fillet, fresh or frozen

- Olive oil cooking spray

- Chopped fresh parsley and lemon wedges for garnish

Preparation:

1. Firstly, preheat oven to 425 degrees F. Line a large rimmed baking sheet with parchment paper.

2. Mix mustard, garlic, lemon zest, lemon juice, rosemary, honey, salt and crushed red pepper in a small bowl. Add panko, walnuts and oil in another small bowl.

3. Put the salmon on the prepared baking sheet. Put the mustard mixture over the fish and sprinkle with the panko mixture, pressing to adhere. Lightly coat with cooking spray.

4. Start baking until the fish flakes easily with a fork, about 8 to 12 minutes, depending on thickness.

5. Scatter parsley and serve with lemon wedges, if desired.

Turmeric chicken noodle soup recipe with noodles

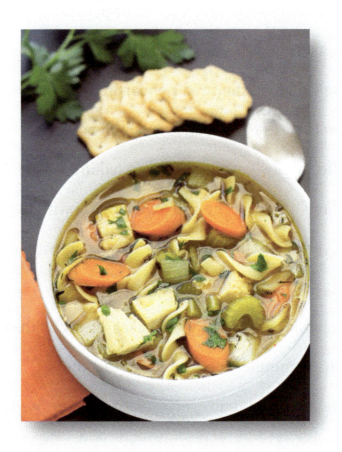

Prep Time: 1 h

Cook Time: 30 min

Serve: 2

Ingredients:

- 1 lb. chicken breast

- cups chopped celery (stem only)

- cups diced carrots

- Salt and pepper

- 1 large onion, diced

- large zucchinis, julienned into thin noodles

- 1 T ground turmeric

- Fresh parsley, to garnish

Preparation:

1. Put chicken breast, diced onions, chopped celery, and diced carrots in a large pot. Cover with water and bring to a boil, then cook until chicken breast is cooked through (about 30 minutes). Chicken is cooked when the juices run clear when you slice into it.

2. Now, transfer the chicken to a plate and let it cool before shredding it into pieces. Add ground turmeric to the soup, then turn heat down to medium-low. Let it simmer for 20 minutes until vegetables are soft. Put in zucchini noodles and cook for 5 minutes.

3. Divide zucchini noodles and soup into two bowls. Top with shredded chicken and garnish using fresh parsley.

Paleo vegan BBQ meatballs

Prep Time: 55 min

Cook Time: 0 min

Serve: 24

Ingredients:

- tablespoon grapeseed oil

- 1 eggplant, skin on, diced

- 1 zucchini, diced

- 1 bell pepper, any color

- ½ cup walnuts, diced very fine

- 1/2 cup paleo BBQ sauce

Preparation:

1. Take a baking sheet out with parchment paper and preheat oven to 350 degrees. In a large pan, heat grapeseed oil. Add pepper, eggplant, walnuts and zucchini.

2. Sautee until browned, for about 15 minutes. Stirring regularly to prevent burning. Remove from heat and let cool for about 5 minutes.

3. Now, add to vitamin blender with tamper and grind until soft- making sure to use tamper to stir mixture. Remove your mixture from blender and put into a larger bowl.

4. After that, take 1/4 cup mixture and roll into a tightly packed ball. Place on parchment paper lined baking sheet. Continue rolling balls. Bake at 350 degrees for 20 minutes, until they're deep brown. This step helps the meatballs "set", so don't skip it!

5. At this time, you can remove your meatballs and freeze them for another use. If eating immediately, place meatballs in a pan with a drizzle of grapeseed oil over medium heat. Brown on all sides, for about 8 minutes.

6. Mix BBQ sauce, stir well. Let sauce heat up- about 2 minutes. Remove from heat and serve immediate.

Turmeric sautéed greens

Prep Time: 3 min

Cook Time: 0 min

Serve: 3-4

Ingredients:

- 1 tablespoon olive oil

- 1 2-inch piece fresh turmeric

- 1/4 teaspoon kosher salt garlic cloves, minced

- tablespoons water

- bunches kale, spinach, or Swiss chard, thinly sliced

Preparation:

1. Firstly, heat oil in a large sauce pan by using medium heat. Now, add garlic and turmeric and sauté for 30 seconds. Further, add kale and salt and sauté for 1 minute.

2. Finally, add water to the pan and cook stirring until the greens are just wilted and serve.

Cauliflower rice

Prep Time: 15 min

Cook Time: 5 min

Serve: 1

Ingredients:

- tablespoons olive oil

- 1 yellow or orange bell pepper

- 1 head cauliflower

- 1 onion, finely diced

- 2 cups fresh spinach, roughly chopped

- 1 cup shelled edamame

- 1/2 teaspoon kosher salt

- teaspoons fresh ginger, minced

- tablespoons low sodium soy sauce scallions, chopped

Preparation:

1. Firstly, heat a large wok or sauté pan over medium heat, add oil and sauté onion and ginger for 1 minute. Put bell pepper and cook for 1 minute.

2. Now, add the cauliflower and cook for an additional 2-3 minutes. Add spinach, edamame, soy sauce and salt. Cook for 4 minutes until the cauliflower is tender.

3. Finely, top with chopped scallions and serve.

Seafood stew

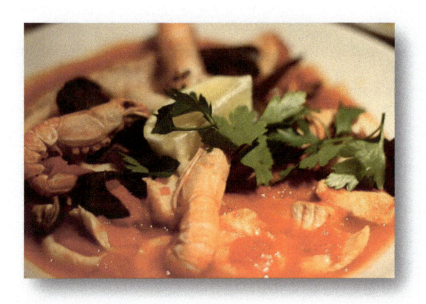

Prep Time: 40 min

Cook Time: 30 min

Serve: 4-6

Ingredients:

- 1 tablespoon oil garlic cloves, minced

- 1 teaspoon kosher salt

- 1 cup dry white wine

- 1 large onion, diced

- 1 bay leaf

- 1 28-ounce can dice tomatoes

- 1/2-pound clams

- 1/2-pound shrimp, peeled and deveined

- 1/2-pound shrimp, peeled and deveined

- 1 cup clam juice

- 1/2-pound mussels

- 1/4 cup minced parsley (optional)

Preparation:

1. Take a large pot, heat oil by using medium heat. Put the onions and cook for 3-4 minutes, until tender. Add garlic and sauté for another minute.

2. Now, add the wine, tomatoes, clam juice, bay leaf and salt. Bring to a boil, then reduce heat and simmer for 20 minutes. Further, put in all the seafood at once and stir. Cook until the shrimp is pink and mussels and clams have opened, about 5-7 minutes.

3. Finely, Garnish with parsley if desired and serve immediately.

Sautéed collard greens

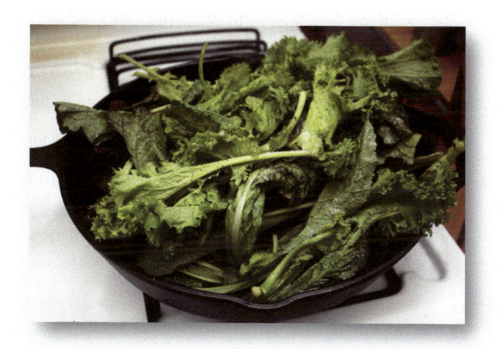

Prep Time: 20 min

Cook Time: 20 min

Serve: 4

Ingredients:

- 1 slice thick-cut bacon, diced

- 1 bunch collard greens garlic cloves, minced

- 1/2 teaspoon kosher salt

Preparation:

1. Firstly, Put the bacon in a pan over medium-low heat and cook for 5 minutes. Remove the stems from the collard greens, and thinly slice the leaves.

2. Now, add the garlic to the pan and cook for 1 minute more. Add the greens and salt and reduce heat to low. Then cook for 5 minutes. Stir when needed. If you like them softer, cook for 10 minutes.

Roasted brussels sprouts with turmeric and mustard seeds

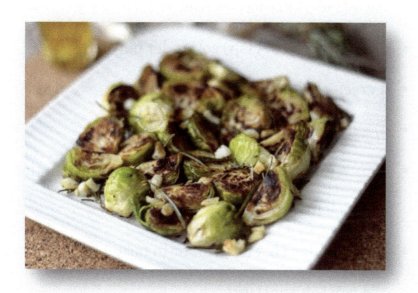

Prep Time: 30 min

Cook Time: 20 min

Serve: 2

Ingredients:

- 1 teaspoon oil

- 1/2 teaspoon (0.5 tsp) black mustard seeds

- 1/4 teaspoon (0.25 tsp) turmeric

- cloves of garlic finely chopped teaspoon or more sesame seeds

- cups (176 g) Brussels sprouts

- 1/2 teaspoon (0.5 tsp) coriander powder

- 1 green chili finely chopped

- 1/2 teaspoon (0.5 tsp) cumin seeds

- 1/2 teaspoon (0.5 tsp) garam masala optional cayenne to taste

- 1/2 teaspoon (0.5 tsp) salt or to taste

- 1/4 cup (62.5 ml) water

- cilantro and lemon for garnish

Preparation:

1. Heat oil in a large skillet. When hot, put cumin and mustard seeds and cook until they change color or start to pop. Further, put curry leaves, garlic and chili carefully. Cook for a minute. Now, add Brussels sprouts.

2. Cook for 5 minutes until some edges get golden brown. Stir when needed. Put sesame seeds, mix in and cook for a minute. Mix in ground spices, salt and mix in and cook for a minute.

3. Add water. Cover and cook for 7 to 9 minute to steam the sprouts. Finely, adjust salt. Add some lemon and cilantro and serve.

Avocado egg boats

Prep Time: 40min

Cook Time: 8 min

Serve: 4

Ingredients:

- Freshly ground black pepper

- ripe avocados, halved and pitted slices bacon

- large eggs

- Kosher salt

- Freshly chopped chives, for garnish

Preparation:

1. Firstly, preheat oven to 350°. Scoop about 1 tbsp. worth of avocado out of each half;

2. Put hollowed avocados in a baking dish, then crack eggs into a bowl, one at a time. Use a spoon, transfer one yolk to each avocado half, and then spoon in as much egg white as you can fit.

3. Add in salt and pepper and bake until whites are set and yolks are no longer runny, 20 to 25 minutes. (Cover with foil if avocados are beginning to brown.)

4. In the meantime, in a large skillet over medium heat, cook bacon until crisp, 8 minutes, and then transfer to a paper towel-lined plate and chop. Finally, top avocados with bacon and chives before serving.

Stuffed Mushrooms

Prep Time: 10 min

Cook Time: 20 min

Serve: 3

Ingredients:

- 20 large mushrooms, washed

- 1 tbsp. extra virgin olive oil

- 1 cup broccoli, chopped

- 1 medium red onion, diced

- 1 tsp. Garlic, minced

- ¼ cup capers

- ½ tsp. Dried oregano

- ½ tsp. dried parsley

- tbsp. feta cheese

- 1 tbsp. breadcrumbs

- Salt and pepper to taste

Preparation:

1. Preheat oven to 425 ° F. Remove the stems from the mushrooms carefully and dice them.

2. Place mushroom tops in a single layer on a baking sheet, with the hole facing up, and bake for 5 minutes.

3. Put olive oil in a pan with the diced mushrooms stems, broccoli, onion, garlic, capers, oregano, parsley and salt, and pepper. Cook for 7 minutes. Add feta and breadcrumbs.

4. Stuff mushrooms with mixture and bake for 8 minutes.

Kale with Pine Nuts

Prep Time: 10 min

Cook Time: 10 min

Serve: 4

Ingredients:

- 1 tbsp. olive oil garlic cloves, minced

- 1½ lb. fresh kale, tough ribs removed and chopped

- ¼ cup water

- tsp. red wine vinegar

- Salt and add black pepper, to taste

- 1 tbsp. pine nuts

Preparation:

1. Heat the olive oil in a large wok over medium heat and sauté the garlic for about 1 minute. Add the kale and cook for 4 minutes.

2. Add the water, vinegar, salt, and black pepper and cook for 5 minutes. Remove from heat and stir in the pine nuts.

3. Serve immediately.

Buckwheat Tuna Casserole

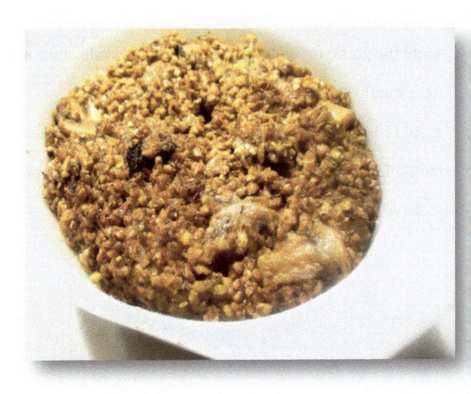

Prep Time: 10 min

Cook Time: 35 min

Serve: 2

Ingredients:

- tbsp. butter

- 10- oz. package buckwheat ramen noodles cups boiling water

- 1/3 cup dry red wine

- cups of milk

- tbsp. dried parsley

- tsp. Turmeric

- ½ tsp. curry powder

- tbsp. all-Purpose flour cups celery, chopped

- 1 cup frozen peas cans tuna, drained

Preparation:

1. Grease your pot with butter. Place buckwheat ramen noodles in a large bowl and pour boiling water to cover.

2. Let it sit for 7 minutes, or until noodles separate when prodded with a fork. In a separate bowl, whisk together red wine, milk, parsley, turmeric, and flour.

3. Fold in celery, peas, and tuna. Drain the ramen and place it into the crockpot, pouring the tuna mixture over the top.

4. Mix to combine. Cover and cook for an hour, stirring occasionally.

Thyme Mushrooms

Prep Time: 10 min

Cook Time: 30 min

Serve: 2

Ingredients:

- 1 tbsp. chopped thyme

- tbsps... olive oil

- tbsps... chopped parsley minced garlic cloves

- Salt and black pepper to taste

- lbs. halved white mushrooms

Preparation:

1. In a baking pan, combine the mushrooms with the garlic and the other ingredients, toss, introduce in the oven and cook at 400°F for 30 minutes.

2. Divide between plates and serve.

Scallops with Mushrooms

Prep Time: 5 min

Cook Time: 10 min

Serve: 4

Ingredients:

- 1 lb. scallops

- tbsp. olive oil

- scallions, chopped

- ½ cup mushrooms, sliced

- tbsp. almonds, chopped

- cup coconut cream

Preparation:

1. Heat a pan with the oil over medium heat; add the scallions and the mushrooms and sauté for 2 minutes.

2. Add the scallops cook over medium heat for 8 minutes more, divide into bowls and serve.

Courgette Risotto

Prep Time: 10 min

Cook Time: 8 min

Serve: 8

Ingredients:

- tbsp. olive oil

- cloves garlic, finely chopped

- lb. Arborio rice

- tomatoes, chopped

- tsp. chopped rosemary

- courgettes, finely diced

- 1 ¼ cups peas, fresh or frozen cups hot vegetable stock

- 1 cup chopped

- Salt and ground

- black pepper to taste

Preparation:

1. Place a large, heavy-bottomed pan over medium heat. Add oil. When the oil is heated, add onion and sauté until translucent.

2. Stir in the tomatoes and cook until soft. Next, stir in the rice and rosemary. Mix well. Add half the stock and cook until dry. Stir frequently.

3. Add remaining stock and cook for 3-4 minutes. Add courgette and peas and cook until rice is tender. Add salt and pepper to taste. Stir in the basil and let it sit for 5 minutes.

4. Serve warm and enjoy

Braised Leek with Pine Nuts

Prep Time: 45 min

Cook Time: 15 min

Serve: 2

Ingredients:

- tbsp. Ghee

- tsp Olive oil pieces Leek

- oz. Vegetable broth

- A bunch of fresh parsley

- 1 tbsp. fresh oregano

- 1 tbsp. Pine nuts (roasted)

Preparation:

1. Cut the leek into thin rings and finely chop the herbs. Roast the pine nuts in a dry pan over medium heat.

2. Melt the ghee together with the olive oil in a large pan. Cook the leek until golden brown for 5 minutes, stirring constantly.

3. Add the vegetable broth and cook for another 10 minutes until the leek is tender. Stir in the herbs and sprinkle the pine nuts on the dish just before serving.

Parsley Butter Shrimp

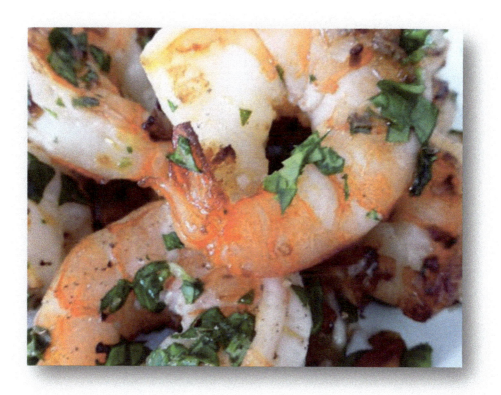

Prep Time: 10 min

Cook Time: 22 min

Serve: 4

Ingredients:

- 1 lb. shrimp, peeled and deveined

- tbsp. butter, divided

- cloves garlic, minced
- ½ cup chicken stock
- tbsp. parsley, minced
- tbsp. Lemon juice
- ¼ tsp. Red pepper flakes
- ½ tsp. Black pepper
- ½ tsp. kosher salt

Preparation:

1. Heat 2 tbsp. of butter in a large, heavy-bottomed skillet over medium heat. Add the shrimp to the skillet and sprinkle with salt and pepper.

2. Cook, occasionally stirring, for 5 minutes or until shrimp is cooked through. Remove shrimp to a plate and set aside.

3. Add the garlic to the skillet and cook, constantly stirring, for 30 seconds. Add the chicken stock and whisk to combine. Simmer until the stock has reduced by half, about 7 minutes.

4. Add the remaining 4 tbsp. of butter, lemon juice, and red pepper to the sauce. Stir to melt the butter and cook for two more minutes.

5. Remove from heat and return the shrimp to the sauce. Sprinkle the parsley over the top and stir to combine. Serve immediately.

Foil Baked Salmon

Prep Time: 8 min

Cook Time: 20 min

Serve: 2

Ingredients:

- salmon fillets
- asparagus spears
- 1 tsp. dried oregano
- slices onion
- 1 tsp. fresh parsley, chopped
- slices lemon
- 1 tbsp. extra virgin olive oil
- Salt and black pepper to taste

Preparation:

1. Preheat oven to 400° F. In a medium bowl, place the two pieces of salmon. Pour 1 tbsp. Of olive oil and sprinkle salt, pepper, and dried oregano.

2. Cut two sheets of foil. It has to be big enough to wrap the salmon and asparagus. First place asparagus, about 8 spears, on the sheet of foil. Layer fillets over asparagus, then top each with about two onion slices and two lemon slices.

3. Wrap sides of foil inward over salmon, fold on top and bottom of the foil to enclose. Place foil packets in a single layer on a baking sheet.

4. Bake in preheated oven for about 15 minutes. Unwrap and using a large spatula, transfer the foil packets to plates. Serve warm!

Baked Zesty Tilapia

Prep Time: 10 min

Cook Time: 10 min

Serve: 4

Ingredients:

- tilapia fillets

- ¼ cup unsalted butter, melted cloves

- garlic, minced

- tbsp. freshly squeezed lemon juice to taste

- Zest of 1 lemon

- tbsp. chopped fresh parsley leaves

- Kosher salt and black pepper to taste

Preparation:

1. Preheat the oven to 425° F. Lightly grease a baking dish or coat with non-stick spray. In a small bowl, whisk together butter, lemon juice, garlic, and lemon zest and set aside.

2. Season the fillets with salt and pepper, taste and place onto the prepared baking dish and drizzle with butter mixture.

3. Place into the oven and bake until fish flakes easily with a fork, about 10 minutes. Serve immediately, garnished with parsley.

Prawns with Asparagus

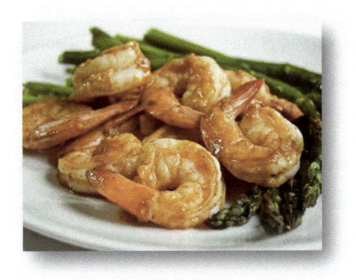

Prep Time: 10 min

Cook Time: 12 min

Serve: 4

Ingredients:

- tbsp. olive oil

- 1 lb. prawns, peeled, and deveined

- 1 lb. asparagus, trimmed

- Salt and black pepper, to taste

- 1 tsp. garlic, minced

- 1 tsp. fresh ginger, minced

- 1 tbsp. low-sodium soy sauce

- tbsp. lemon juice

Preparation:

1. In a wok, heat 2 tbsp. of oil over medium-high heat and cook the prawns with salt and black pepper for about 4 minutes. With a slotted spoon, transfer the prawns into a bowl and set aside.

2. In the same wok, heat remaining 1 tbsp. Of oil over medium-high heat and cook the asparagus, ginger, garlic, salt, and black pepper and sauté for about 7 minutes, stirring frequently. Stir in the prawns and soy sauce and cook for about 1 minute.

3. Stir in the lemon juice and remove from the heat. Serve hot.

Tuna and Kale

Prep Time: 5 min

Cook Time: 20 min

Serve: 4

Ingredients:

- 1 lb. tuna fillets, boneless, skinless and cubed

- tbsp. olive oil

- 1 cup kale, torn

- ½ cup cherry tomatoes, cubed

- 1 yellow onion, chopped

Preparation:

1. Heat a pan with the oil over medium heat. Add the onion and sauté for 5 minutes. Add the tuna and the other ingredients.

2. Toss and cook everything for 15 minutes more, divide between plates and serve.

Minty Soup

Prep and Cook Time: 35 min

Serve: 6

Ingredients:

- chopped garlic cloves – 2

- water – 1 cup

- olive oil – 2 tbsps

- heavy cream – ¼ cup

- vegetable stock – 2 cups

- chopped shallots - 2

- lemon juice – 1 tbsp

- chopped mint leaves - 4

- dried oregano – ½ tsp

- Pepper and salt to taste

- pound green peas - 1

Preparation:

1. In garlic and shallots, stir heated oil in a soup pot and cook until it's softened for 2 minutes. Then add oregano, green peas, stock, mint and water.

2. Cook for 15 minutes on a low heat after adding pepper and salt to taste. In the lemon juice, stir and cook it for 2 more minutes.

3. Remove from heat when it is done and stir it in the cream. Use an immersion blender to puree the soup immersion blender until it is smooth and creamy. Best served chilled or warm.

Special Orzo Soup

Cook and Prep Time: 45 min

Serve: 8

Ingredients:

- Orzo – ¼ cup

- vegetable stock – 2 cups

- lemon juice – 2 tbsps

- cored and diced yellow bell pepper - 1

- extra virgin olive oil – 2 tbsps

- chopped shallots - 2

- baby spinach – 4 cups

- green peas – 1 cup

- cored and diced green bell pepper - 1

- water – 4 cups

- chopped garlic cloves - 2

- Pepper and salt to taste

Preparation:

1. In a soup pot, heat the oil and stir in the garlic and shallots. Add other Ingredients: after cooking it for 2 minutes and season with pepper and salt.

2. On low heat, cook it for 25 minutes. Best served chilled or warm.

Sweet and gorgeous Lentil Stew

Cook and Prep Time: 45 min

Serve: 8

Ingredients:

- water – 3 cups

- crushed tomatoes – 1 can

- extra virgin olive oil – 2 tbsps

- chopped garlic cloves – 2

- diced carrots - 2

- cored and diced red bell peppers - 2

- diced celery stalk – 1

- cumin seeds – ½ tsp

- mustard seeds – ½ tsp

- chopped shallots - 2

- vegetable stock – 3 cups

- Pepper and salt to taste

- green lentils – 1 cup

- Yogurt for serving

Preparation:

1. In a soup pot, heat the oil and stir in the garlic and shallots. Add other Ingredients: after cooking it for 2 minutes. On low heat, adjust the taste with pepper and salt for 30 minutes.

2. Top it with freshly chopped parsley or plain yogurt after serving the soup fresh and warm.

Delicious Meatball Soup for the Spanish

Cook and Prep Time: 1 h

Serve: 8

Ingredients:

- water – 6 cups

- crushed tomatoes – 1 can

- egg - 1

- olive oil – 2 tbsps

- diced celery stalk - 1

- chopped onion - 1

- cored and diced red bell peppers – 2

- vegetable stock – 2 cups

- diced carrots - 2

- pound ground veal - 1

- chopped parsley – 2 tbsps

- chopped garlic cloves - 2

- Pepper and salt to taste

Preparation:

1. In a soup pot, heat the oil and stir in the garlic, stock, bell peppers, onions, carrots, water and celery. Bring to a boiling after seasoning with pepper and salt.

2. In a bowl, mix egg, veal and parsley in the meantime. Then boil them in boiling liquid after forming small meatballs. Adjust the taste with pepper and salt after adding the tomatoes. For 20 minutes, cook on very low heat. Best served fresh and warm.

Rice Rolls

Prep Time: 15 min

Cook Time: 35 min

Serve: 6

Ingredients:

- 4 white cabbage leaves

- 4 oz ground chicken

- ½ tsp. garlic powder

- ¼ cup of long grain rice, cooked

- ½ cup chicken stock

- ½ cup tomatoes, chopped

Preparation:

1. In the bowl, mix ground chicken, garlic powder, and rice.

2. Then put the rice mixture on every cabbage leaf and roll.

3. Arrange the rice rolls in the saucepan. Add chicken stock and tomatoes and close the lid.

4. Cook the rice rolls for 35 minutes on low heat.

Rice Stew with Squid

Prep Time: 10 min

Cook Time: 30 min

Serve: 6

Ingredients:

- 5 oz long grain rice

- 4 oz squid, sliced

- 1 jalapeno pepper, chopped

- ½ cup tomatoes, chopped

- 1 onion, diced

- 2 cups chicken stock

- 1 tbsp. avocado oil

Preparation:

1. Roast the onion with avocado oil in the skillet for 3-4 minutes or until the onion is light brown. Add squid, jalapeno pepper, and tomatoes. Cook the ingredients for 7 minutes. Then cook rice with water for 15 minutes.

2. Add cooked rice in the squid mixture, stir, and cook for 3 minutes more.

Creamy Millet

Prep Time: 10 min

Cook Time: 10 min

Serve: 6

Ingredients:

- ½ cup millet

- 1 oz cream cheese

- ¼ tsp. salt

- 1.5 cup hot water

Preparation:

Mix hot water and millet in the saucepan. Boil it for 8 minutes on low heat. Add cream cheese and salt. Carefully stir the cooked millet.

Oatmeal Cakes

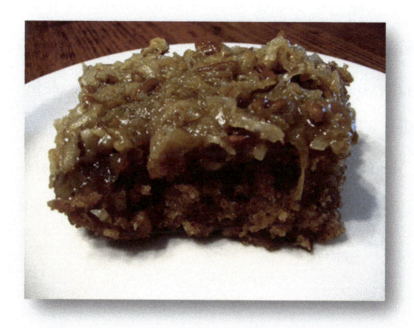

Prep Time: 15 min

Cook Time: 7 min

Serve: 4

Ingredients:

- ½ cup oatmeal

- 1 egg, beaten

- 1 carrot, grated

- 1 tbsp. olive oil

- 1 tsp. flax meal

Preparation

1. Put oatmeal, egg, grated carrot, and flax meal in the blender. Blend the mixture well. Then heat olive oil in the skillet.

2. Make the medium-sized cakes from the oatmeal mixture and cook for 3 minutes per side on medium heat.

Yogurt Buckwheat

Prep Time: 5 min

Cook Time: 13 min

Serve: 2

Ingredients:

- ½ cup buckwheat

- 1.5 cup chicken stock

- 1 tbsp. plain yogurt

Preparation:

Put all ingredients in the saucepan and close the lid. Cook the meal for 13 minutes on low heat or until the buckwheat soaks all liquid. Carefully stir the cooked meal.

Halloumi Buckwheat Bowl

Prep Time: 10 min

Cook Time: 15 min

Serve: 4

Ingredients:

- 1 cup buckwheat

- cups chicken stock

- 4 oz halloumi cheese

- 1 tbsp. olive oil

- ½ tsp. dried thyme

Preparation:

1. Mix chicken stock and buckwheat in the saucepan, boil, and cook for 7 minutes on medium heat. After this, sprinkle the halloumi cheese with olive oil and dried thyme.

2. Grill it for 2 minutes per side or until the cheese is light brown. Then put the cooked buckwheat in the bowls.

3. Chop the cheese roughly and top the buckwheat with it.

Aromatic Green Millet

Prep Time: 10 min

Cook Time: 7 min

Serve: 5

Ingredients:

- 1 cup millet

- 2 cups of water

- 4 tbsp. pesto sauce

- ¼ tsp. cayenne pepper

-

- **Preparation:**

1. Mix water and millet in the saucepan and boil for 7 minutes. Then add cayenne pepper and pesto sauce.

2. Stir the millet until homogenous and green.

Quinoa with Pumpkin

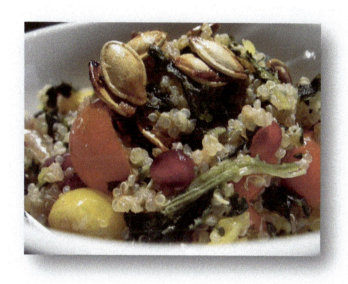

Prep Time: 5 min

Cook Time: 20 min

Serve: 6

Ingredients:

- ½ cup pumpkin, cubed

- 1 tbsp. lemon juice

- 1 tsp. liquid honey

- 1 cup quinoa

- 2 cups of water

- ¼ cup of organic almond milk

Preparation:

1. Put almond milk and pumpkin in the saucepan. Add lemon juice and water. Cook the pumpkin for 10 minutes.

2. Then add quinoa and cook the meal for 10 minutes.

3. Remove the cooked meal from the heat, add liquid honey, and stir well.

Almond Quinoa

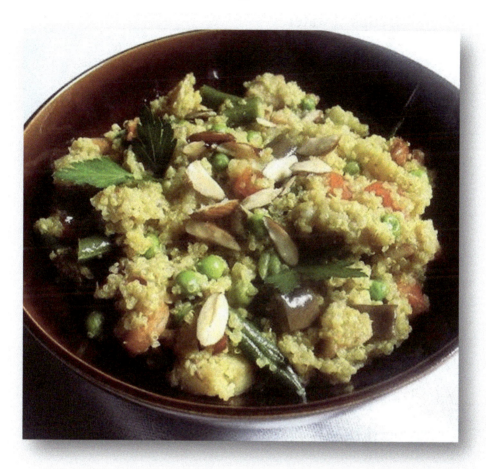

Prep Time: 5 min

Cook Time: 4 min

Serve: 4

Ingredients:

- 1 cup quinoa

- 2 cups of water

- 1 cup organic almond milk

- ½ cup strawberries, sliced

- 1 tbsp. honey

Preparation:

1. Pour water and milk in the saucepan and bring to boil.

2. Add quinoa and cook it for 12 minutes. Then cool the cooked quinoa and add honey. Stir.

3. Transfer the quinoa in the bowls and top with strawberries.

Spring Rolls with Quinoa

Prep Time: 10 min

Cook Time: 1 min

Serve: 8

Ingredients:

- 8 rice pepper wraps

- 1 cup quinoa, cooked

- 1 carrot, cut into strips

- 1 cup lettuce leaves

- 1 tbsp. olive oil

Preparation:

1. Make the rice pepper wraps wet. Then put the cooked quinoa on every rice pepper wrap.

2. Add carrot and lettuce leaves and wrap them into the rolls. Brush every roll with olive oil and put it in the hot skillet. Roast the spring rolls for 20 seconds per side.

Mushroom Quinoa Skillet

Prep Time: 10 min

Cook Time: 25 min

Serve: 6

Ingredients:

- 1 cup mushrooms, sliced

- ½ cup of water

- 1 tbsp. olive oil

- 1 tsp. Italian seasonings

- ½ cup quinoa

- ½ cup organic almond milk

- ¼ tsp. dried thyme

Preparation:

1. Roast mushrooms with olive oil in the saucepan for 10 minutes. Then stir them well, add Italian seasonings, dried thyme, and quinoa.

2. Add almond milk and water.

3. Close the lid and simmer the meal for 15 minutes. Stir it from time to time to avoid burning.

Strawberry Quinoa Bowl

Prep Time: 15 min

Cook Time: 0 min

Serve: 8

Ingredients:

- 2 ½ cup quinoa, cooked

- ¼ cup strawberries, roughly chopped

- ½ cup fresh spinach, chopped

- 2 pecans, chopped

- 1 tbsp. balsamic vinegar

- 1 tsp. avocado oil

Preparation:

1. Mix quinoa, fresh spinach, and pecans in the big bowl.

2. Then add strawberries and avocado oil. Gently shake the mixture and transfer in the serving bowls.

3. Sprinkle every serving with a small amount of balsamic vinegar.

Quinoa Meatballs

Prep Time: 15 min

Cook Time: 30 min

Serve: 6

Ingredients:

- ½ cup quinoa, cooked

- ½ cup ground pork

- 1 tbsp. chives, chopped

- 1 egg, beaten

- 1 tbsp. sesame seeds

- 1 tsp. chili flakes

- 1 cup tomato juice

Preparation:

1. In the bowl mi quinoa, ground pork, chives, egg, sesame seeds, and chili flakes. Then make the small meatballs and put them in the baking pan.

2. Top the meatballs with tomato juice and cook in the preheated to 375F oven for 30 minutes.

Stir-Fried Farro

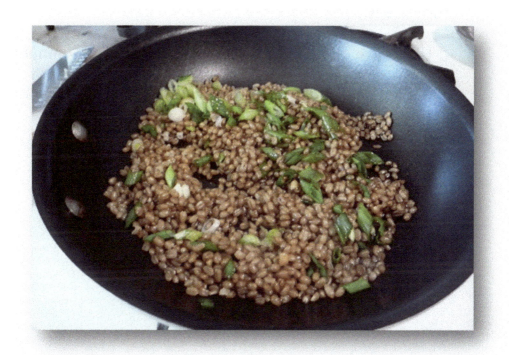

Prep Time: 10 min

Cook Time: 8 min

Serve: 4

Ingredients:

- 1 cup farro, cooked

- 1 egg, beaten

- 1 tbsp. olive oil

- ½ tsp. chili flakes

Preparation:

1. Heat olive oil and egg beaten egg. Cook it for 1 minute and then stir it carefully. Add cooked farro and chili flakes.

2. Fry the meal for 7 minutes. Stir it from time to time.

Quick Farro Skillet

Prep Time: 10 min

Cook Time: 15 min

Serve: 6

Ingredients:

- 2 oz fresh spinach, chopped

- 2 oz asparagus, chopped

- 1/3 cup farro, cooked

- 1 tbsp. olive oil

- ½ tsp. curry powder

Preparation:

Line the skillet with baking paper. Put all ingredients in the prepared skillet, flatten them gently and transfer in the preheated to 365°F oven. Cook the meal for 15 minutes.